AFK
Anatomy For Kids

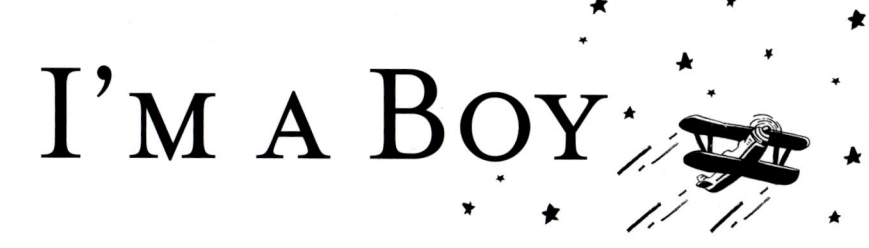

I'm a Boy

My Changing Body
Describes the early signs of puberty

By
Shelley Metten, M.S., Ph.D.
with Alan Estridge

Illustrated By
Maggie Chiang, Jessie Do
& Karen Wang

"Our goal is that children everywhere will have the knowledge to make wise choices in the care of their bodies."
-Dr. Metten, Anatomy for Kids®

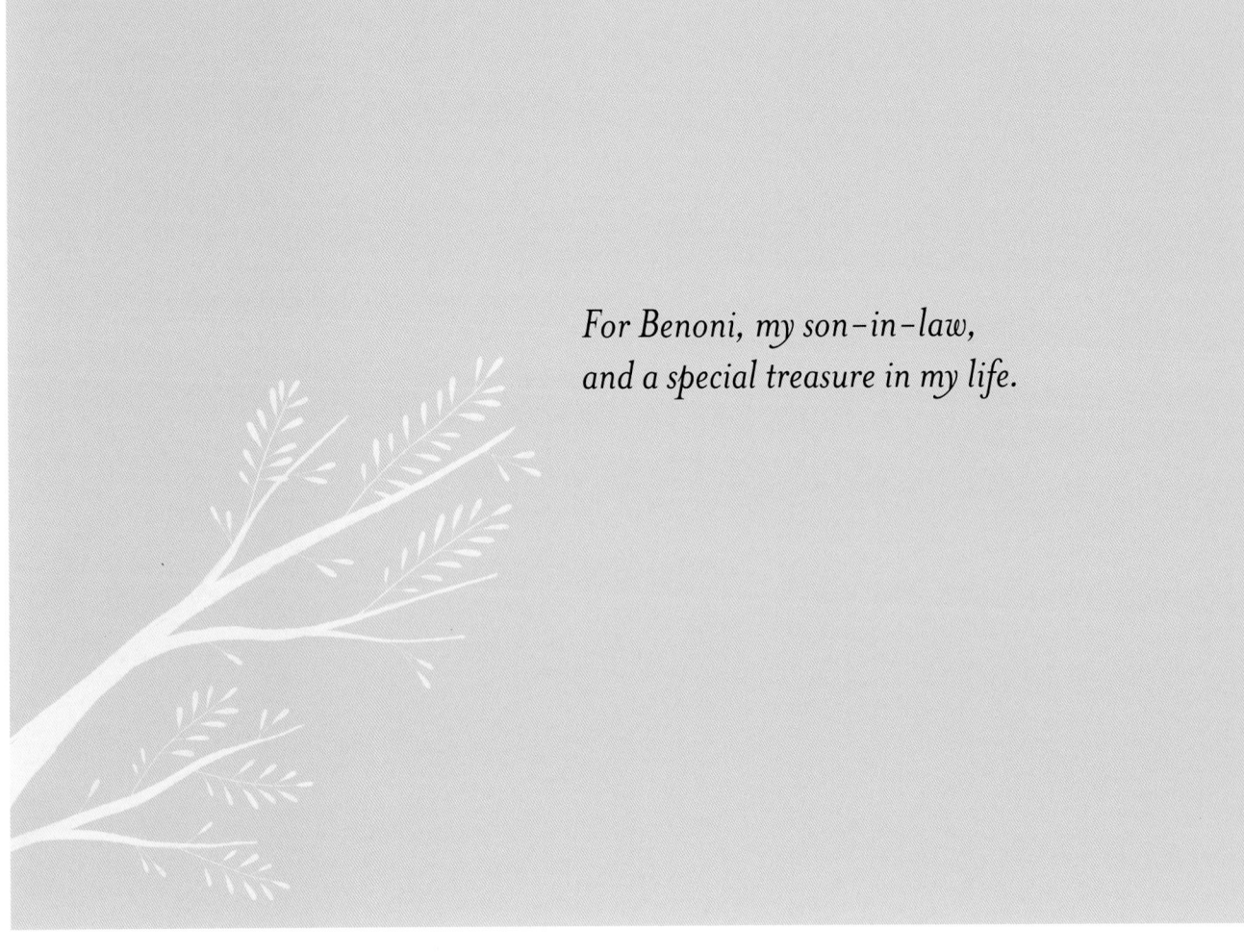

*For Benoni, my son-in-law,
and a special treasure in my life.*

TEXT AND ILLUSTRATIONS COPYRIGHT © 2021 BY ANATOMY FOR KIDS®, LLC

All rights reserved. No part of this book may be reproduced, transmitted, or stored in an information retrieval system in any form or by any means, graphic, electronic, or mechanical, including photocopying, taping, and recording without prior written permission from Anatomy For Kids®, LLC.

ISBN - 13:978-0-9895469-7-3
SECOND EDITION

VISIT US AT WWW.ANATOMYFORKIDS.COM

The information provided in this book is not intended to be a substitute for professional medical advice, diagnosis, or treatment. Always seek the advice of your physician or other qualified health care professional with any questions you may have regarding a medical condition. Reliance on any information provided herein is solely at your own risk.

Reproductive System Series for Boys

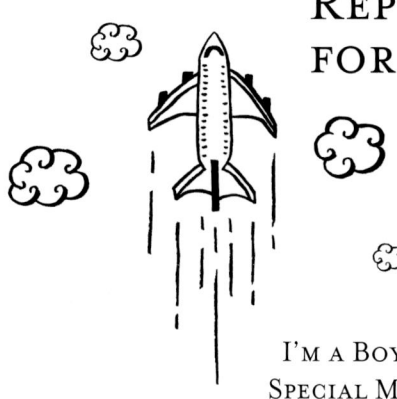

The I'm a Boy Series consists of five books, and provides boys with the knowledge they need to understand the maturing features of their reproductive system. It helps answer the question "why" the changes are happening.

I'm a Boy:
Special Me
(Ages 5-7)

This book is intended to prepare young boys as they enter puberty in just a few years. It introduces the concept that sperm help make babies. It describes the basic structure of the testicles and penis, and also emphasizes the importance for boys to protect their genitals from inappropriate touching.

I'm a Boy:
My Changing Body
(Ages 8-10)

There are two age-appropriate books that describe the changes a boy experiences during puberty. This book is intended for a young boy at the beginning of puberty when he notices changes in his body odor, his skin, and his emotions.

I'm a Boy:
Hormones!
(Ages 11+)

This book describes male reproductive anatomy and the changes that happen later in puberty. It includes information about wet dreams, spontaneous erections, and other changes they are going to experience.

I'm a Boy:
How Are Girls Different?
(Ages 13+)

This book is intended for boys who have learned about the changes in their own body as a result of puberty and want to compare it to the changes happening in a girl's body at a similar age.

I'm a Boy:
Sexual Maturity
(Ages 15+)

This book is intended for boys who are a few years into puberty and who have questions about reproduction. The content addresses conception, contraception, and reproductive health.

Along with the multiple book series, the Anatomy for Kids® website, Facebook page, and YouTube channel provide useful resources to support parents. These learning resources are not intended to promote any specific moral or cultural perspective. Anatomy for Kids® considers that a parent or other concerned adult would prefer to provide that guidance themselves.

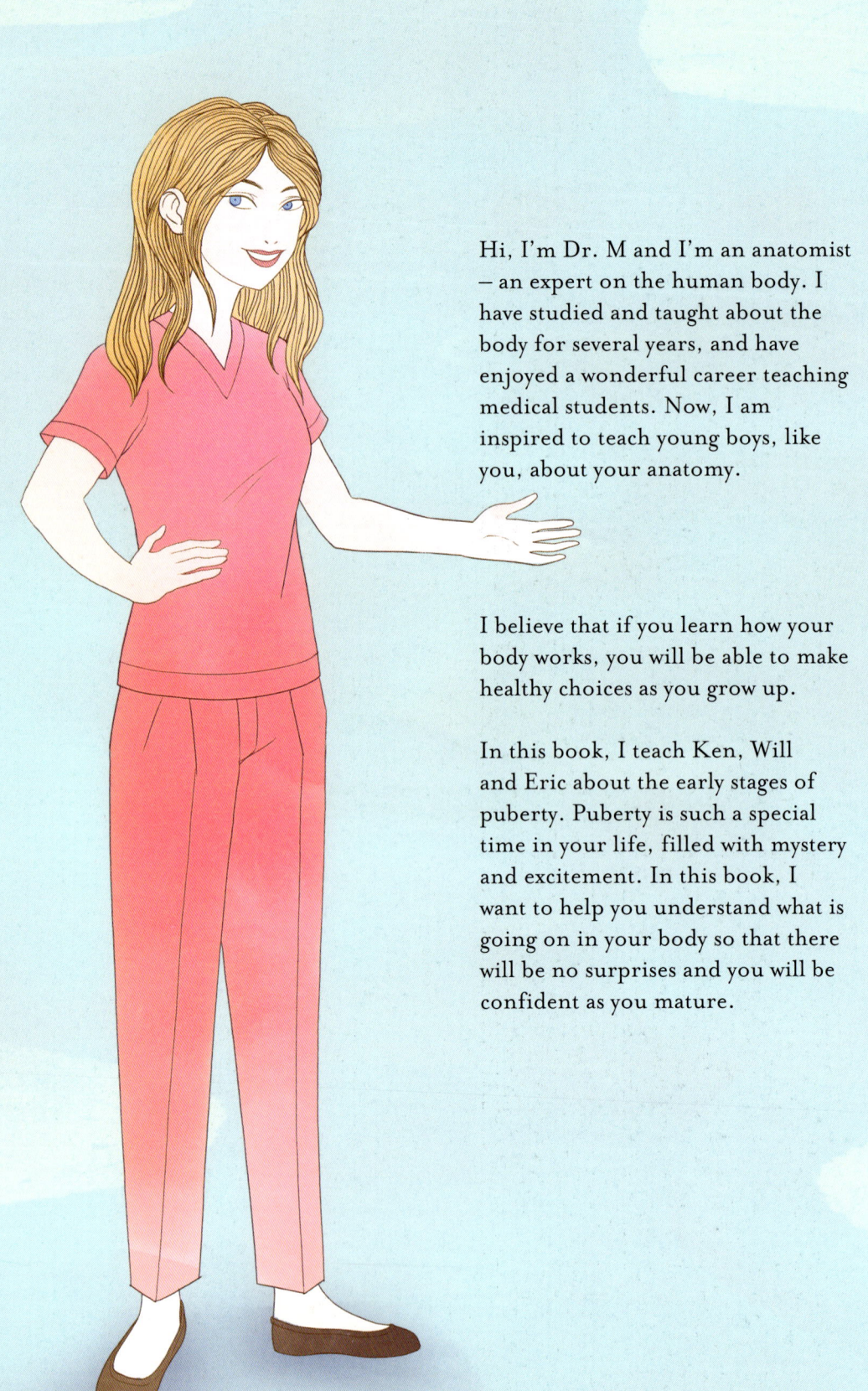

Hi, I'm Dr. M and I'm an anatomist — an expert on the human body. I have studied and taught about the body for several years, and have enjoyed a wonderful career teaching medical students. Now, I am inspired to teach young boys, like you, about your anatomy.

I believe that if you learn how your body works, you will be able to make healthy choices as you grow up.

In this book, I teach Ken, Will and Eric about the early stages of puberty. Puberty is such a special time in your life, filled with mystery and excitement. In this book, I want to help you understand what is going on in your body so that there will be no surprises and you will be confident as you mature.

Looking For Answers?

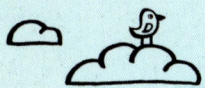

Chapter 1 Puberty	Something is changing down there! What's puberty? How will I know puberty has started?
Chapter 2 Skin Changes	Why do I smell different and have pimples? Why do my breasts hurt and what are pubic hair?
Chapter 3 Genitals	Where is the pelvic cavity? What is inside the penis? Is my penis circumcised? Why does my scrotum look different now?
Chapter 4 Making Sperm	Where are sperm made? What happens to my scrotum when it gets hot or cold? What is inside the testicle? Are my testicles making sperm now?
Chapter 5 Ejaculation	What is ejaculation? How do sperm get from the testicles to the penis? How do sperm get energy? What is semen? Does semen and pee come out the same hole? What's an adolescent?

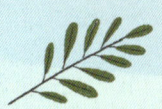

Words in **bold** in the text are defined under **Special Words** on pages 44-45.

Chapter 1

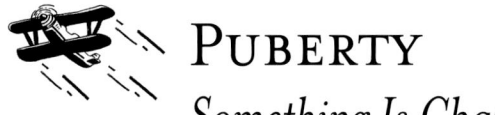

PUBERTY
Something Is Changing Down There!

Ken's dad was helping Ken and his friends pick out new soccer gear. The boys were running around the store looking at all of the equipment. Ken grabbed something off of the rack and held it up to his dad.

"What is this?" asked Ken.

"That's an athletic cup," answered Ken's dad. "It protects your privates from getting hurt."

"You mean our **genitals** (*JIN-uh-tulls*)?" said Eric. "That's what Dr. M said they're called. She told us the genitals are the **scrotum** (*SKRO-tum*) and the **penis**."

"Hey guys," said Will, turning to Ken and Eric. "Have you noticed any changes down there? I think something is happening."

"What do you mean?" asked Eric.

"I don't know what is going on, but I think my scrotum is getting bigger," explained Will.

"Really? Whoa. Maybe we'd better talk to Dr. M again," suggested Ken.

"Boys, I think that's a great idea," said Ken's dad. "I can take you to see her, if it's okay with your parents."

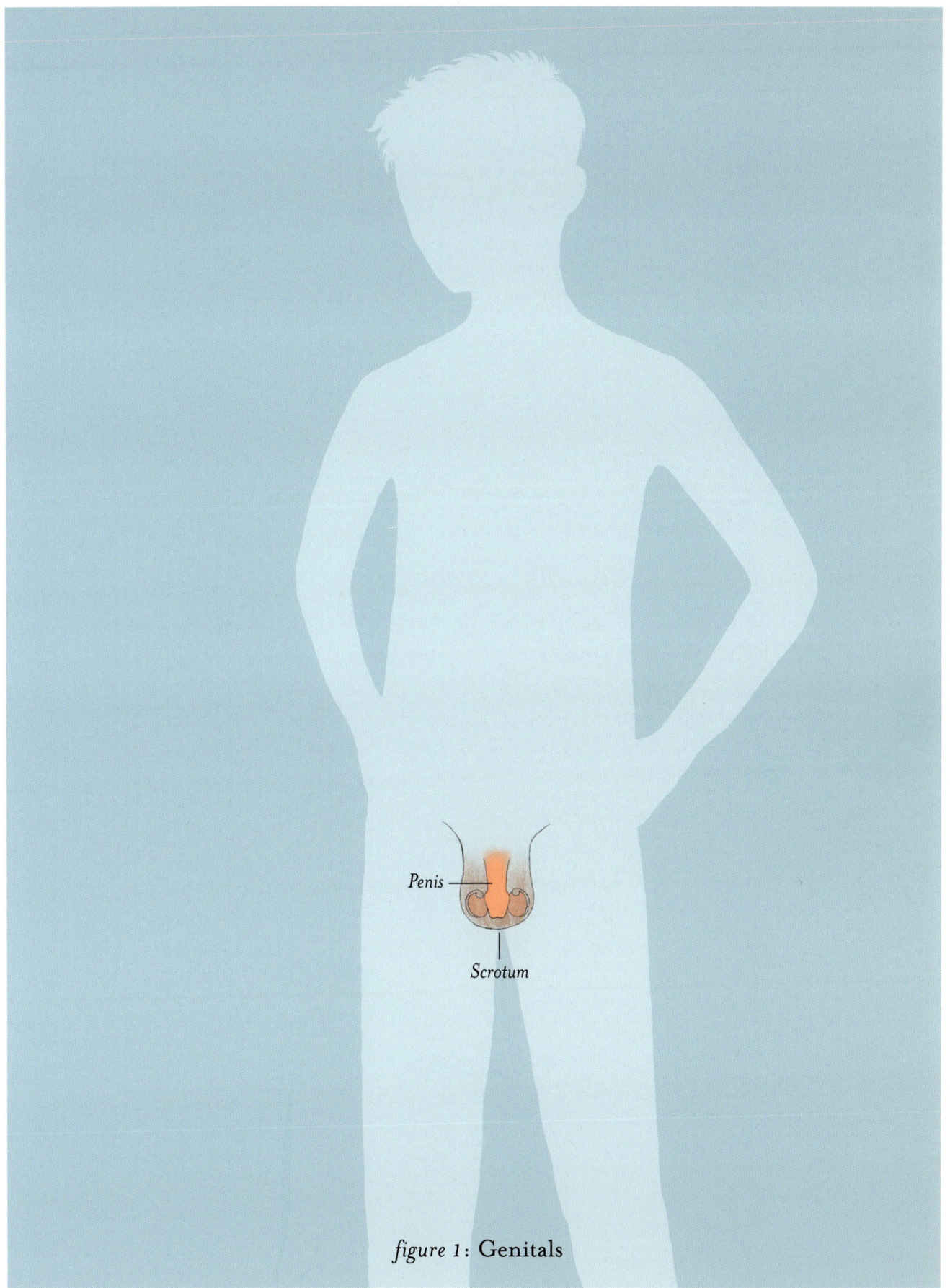

figure 1: Genitals

✦ What's Puberty?

The next day the three boys arrived at Dr. M's office with Ken's dad.

"It's great to see you all again," said Dr. M. "What brings you here today?"

"Well, last time you taught us about our genitals, and now I think something is changing down there," said Will.

"What do you think is changing?" asked Dr. M.

A little embarrassed, Will answered, "I think my scrotum is getting bigger."

"That sounds about right," she responded. "You're starting to see the early signs of **puberty** *(PEW-bur-tee)*."

"Puberty? What's that?" asked Eric.

"Puberty is a time when your reproductive structures are changing," explained Dr. M. "They are maturing so that one day you can help make a baby."

"That doesn't sound right," said Will. "I don't want to help make a baby now!"

"I agree with you, Will," said Dr. M. "You're not ready yet, but it is time for your body to start getting ready."

How Will I Know Puberty Has Started?

Puberty begins very quietly, so you may not even notice it has started. The timing can be different for each boy, but there are some signs as early as nine or ten years old that give you a clue that you have entered the early days of puberty.

Here are a few signs you can look for:

- Something you've probably already noticed is a change in your body odor. Actually, everyone notices that one!

- Slowly there will be changes in your skin as well. Small red bumps called pimples might appear on your face.

- Your scrotum will get a little larger. This isn't a big change in the beginning so you might not see a difference for about a year or more.

- Later on, you will begin to see tiny hairs growing near your genitals.

Dr. M Says:

"There are early signs that let you know you have entered early puberty. Puberty is a time when your body starts making sperm so that one day, when you decide, you can help make a baby."

Chapter 2

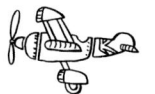 # SKIN CHANGES
Why Do I Smell Different and Have Pimples?

Even at the beginning of puberty, you will notice a change in the way you smell.

"My mom made me start wearing deodorant because the whole family was talking about how bad I smelled!" complained Will.

Dr. M laughed. "Let me tell you something interesting about body odor. Everywhere in your skin are sweat glands. You have already noticed how sweaty you can get after running around outside."

What you might not know is there are bacteria that live on your skin and it is okay for them to be there. In certain places in your body, like your armpits and around your genitals, there are sweat glands that produce a special sweat that the bacteria like. They take in the sweat and produce a smelly gas that is your body odor.

"So, if my body odor changes, I am already starting puberty?" asked Eric.

"That's right Eric, and it seems like all three of you have already experienced the body odor change," observed Dr. M.

Something else you might notice just as puberty starts is a change in the skin on your face. Little red bumps called **pimples** could begin to show up. It is a good idea to keep your face clean and not touch the pimples. They'll come and go over the next few years, but touching them can make the situation worse.

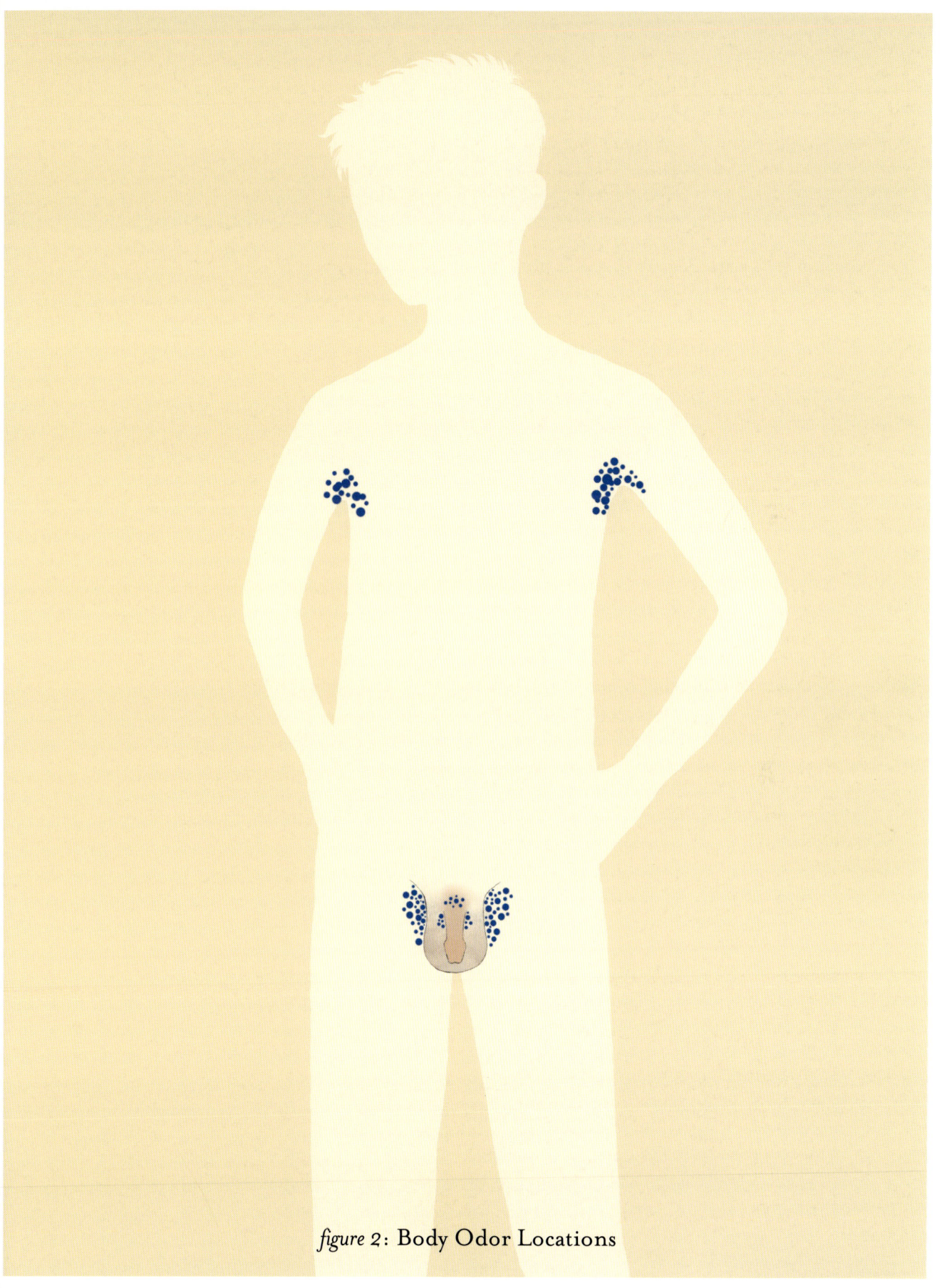

figure 2: Body Odor Locations

Why Do My Breasts Hurt and What Are Pubic Hair?

Another sign that you have started puberty is when you begin to see tiny hairs near your scrotum and penis. They are called **pubic** *(PEW-bic)* **hair**. At first, pubic hair is very thin, but it thickens and becomes curly over the next few years. The special sweat glands that cause body odor are located near pubic hair.

Most boys don't see pubic hair until they are at least 10 years old. In the next few months, you might notice some. But remember, each boy has his own unique experience. You may begin puberty at a different time than your friends. Just know that it will happen for you when your body says the time is right.

There is one more change that most boys experience. One or both of your breasts can feel a little tender for a few months. This is normal for boys during puberty and it won't last too long.

Dr. M Says:

"There are different signs you can see in your skin at the beginning of puberty. There is a change in your body odor and pimples might start showing up on your face. Tiny pubic hair begins to grow near your scrotum and penis. Also, some boys notice that one or both breasts are a little tender for a few months."

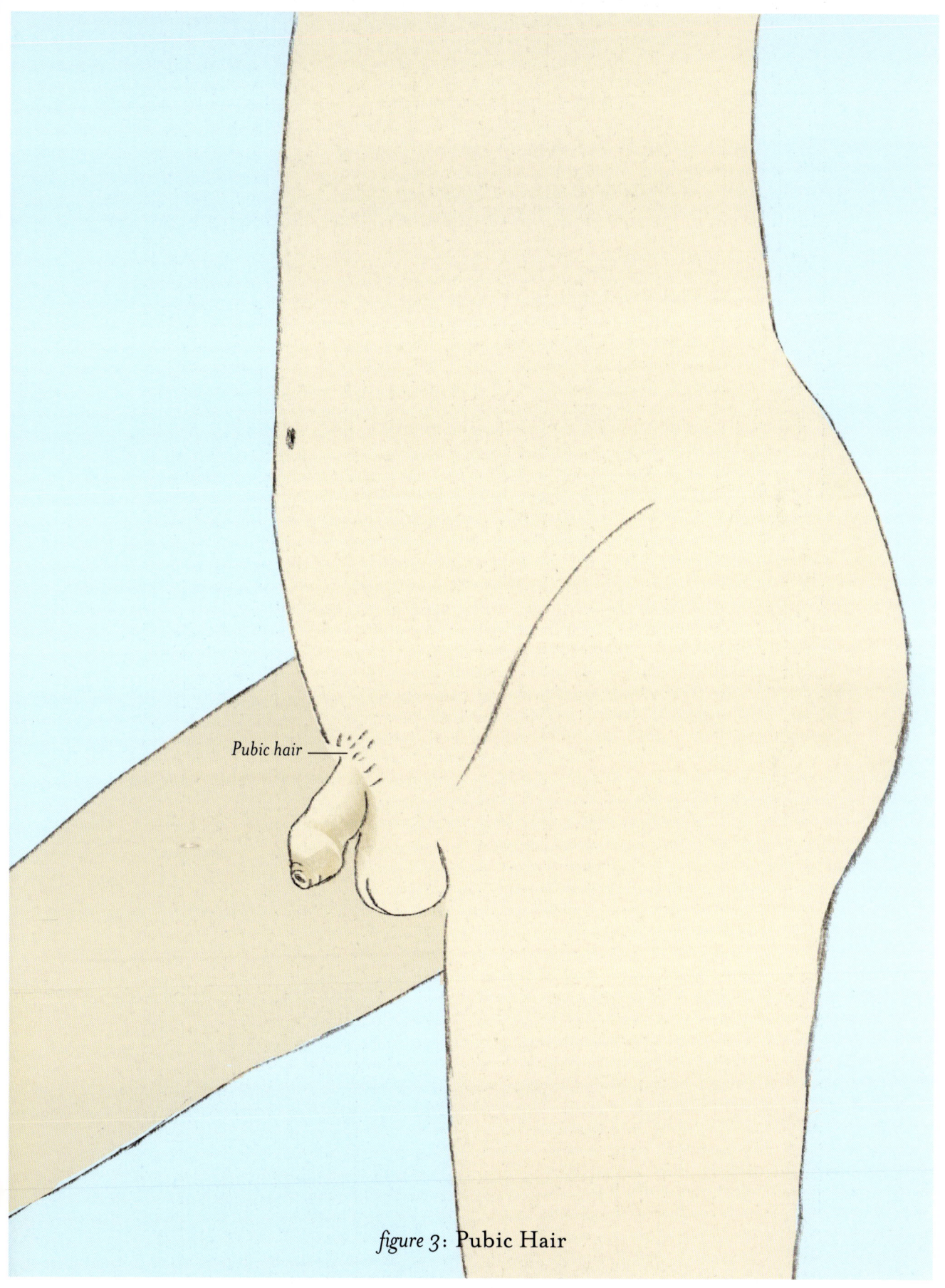

figure 3: Pubic Hair

Chapter 3

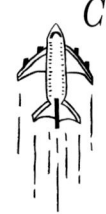

GENITALS
Where is the Pelvic Cavity?

Observe the circle of bone called the **pelvis** in this anatomy figure. If you put your hands on your hips, you are touching the pelvis. There's a space in the center of the pelvis called the **pelvic cavity**.

You have already heard about male reproductive structures that are outside the pelvic cavity. They are the **scrotum** and the **penis**. We call them the genitals.

There are also male reproductive structures that are inside the pelvic cavity. They help make sperm and move them along a path to the penis.

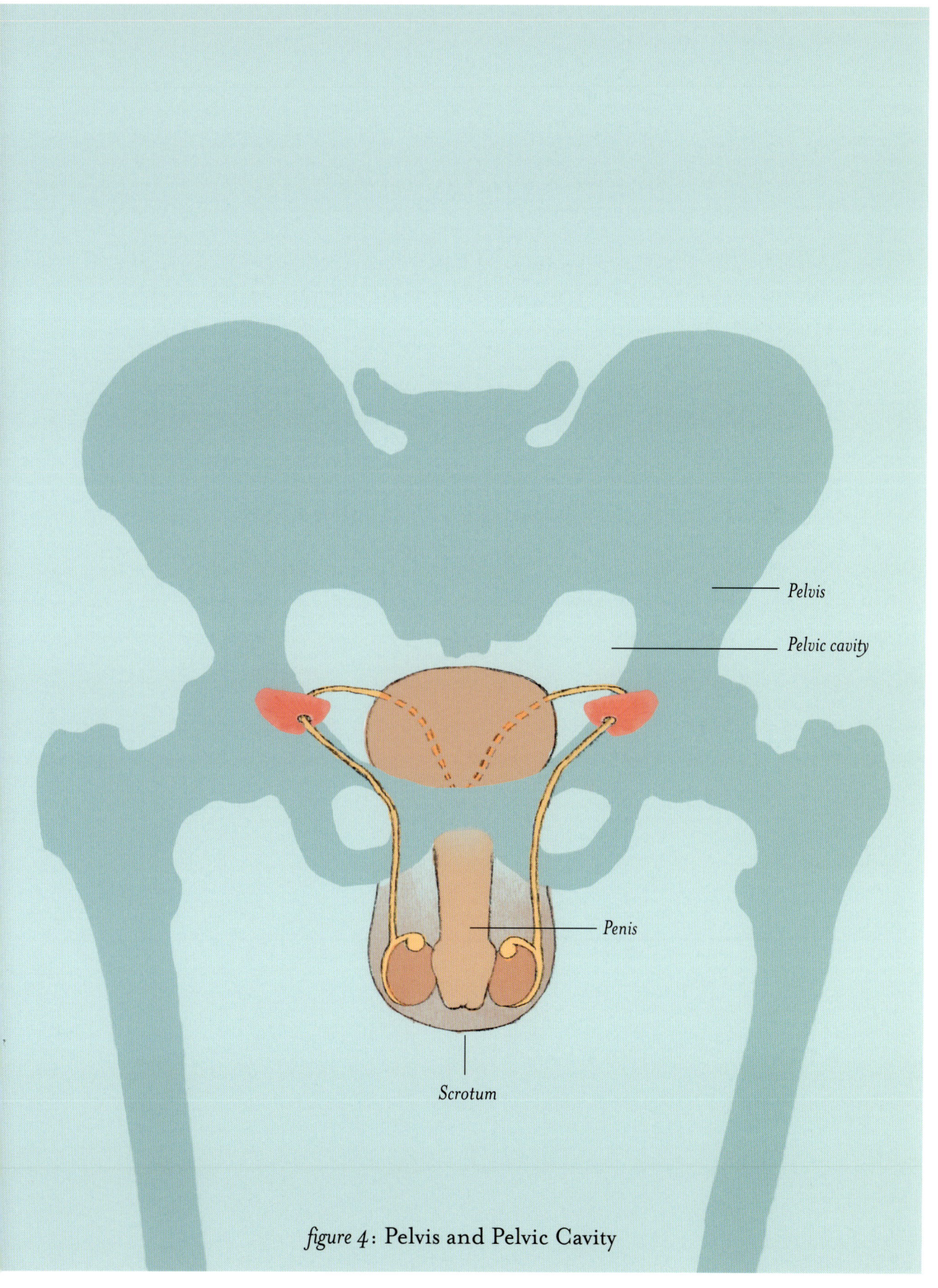

figure 4: Pelvis and Pelvic Cavity

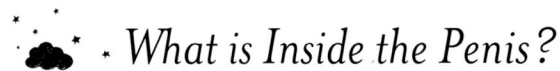 · *What is Inside the Penis?*

Let's talk about the genitals first, starting with the **penis**.

The outside of the penis is covered with skin.

You might be wondering what is inside the penis. The inside of the penis looks like a sponge. In the center of the **spongy part** is a tube called the **urethra** *(you-REE-thruh)*.

Urine, or pee, flows through the urethra and comes out an opening at the end of the penis called the **urethral** *(you-REE-thrul)* **opening**.

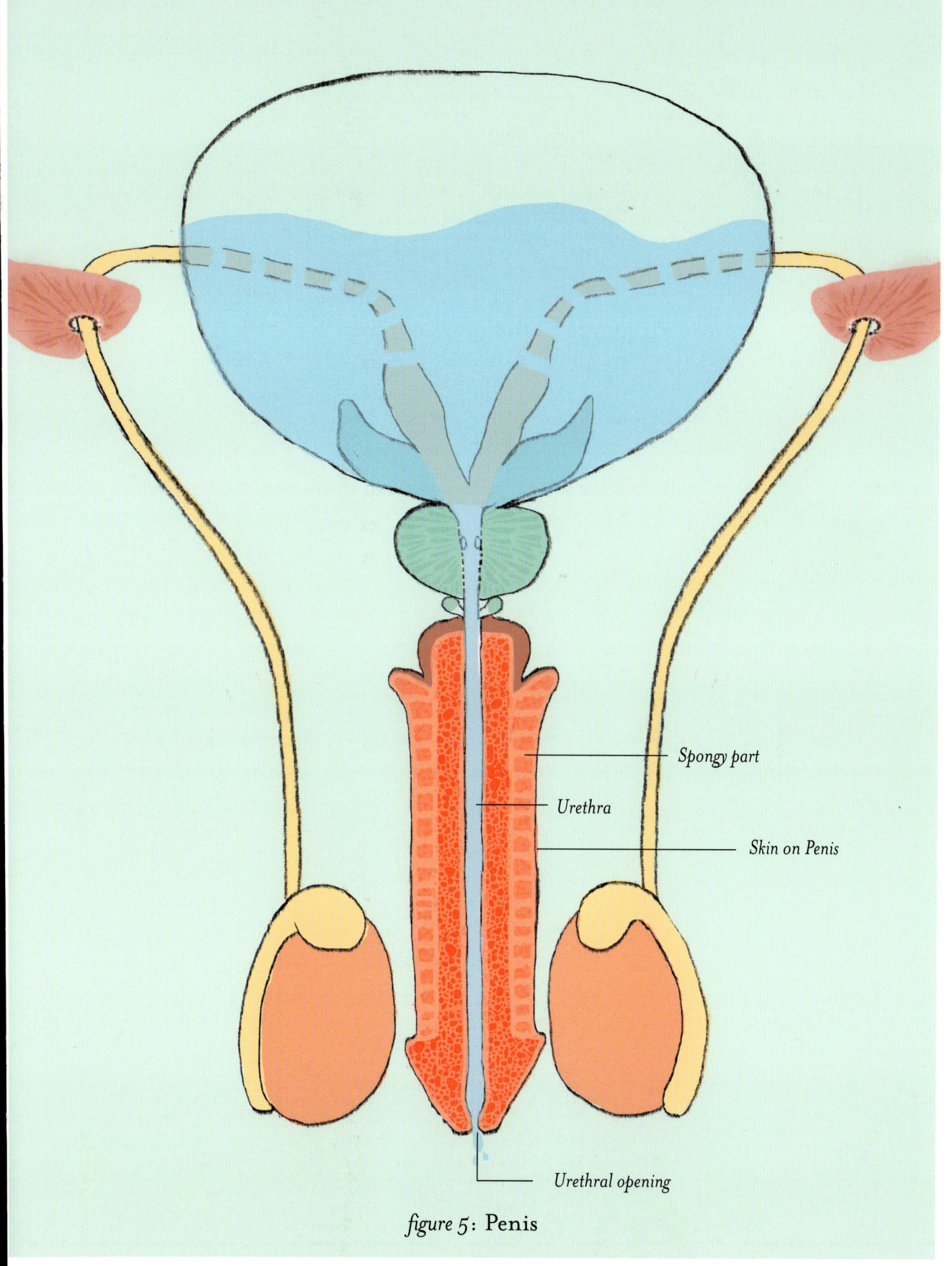

figure 5: Penis

☁ · *Is My Penis Circumcised?*

The end of the penis is called the **glans penis**. The skin on the glans penis folds back and forms a hood that covers the skin on the end of the penis. This hood of skin is called **foreskin**, or **prepuce** *(PRAY-puce)*.

In some boys, when they were a baby, the foreskin was removed in a procedure called **circumcision** *(SIR-kum-si-jun)*. You can see the difference between a **circumcised penis** and an **uncircumcised penis** in these two anatomy figures. Even though the skin on the end of the penis looks different, they function the same.

"So, it doesn't matter which kind of penis we have, or what it looks like?" asked Eric.

"That's right, Eric!" said Dr. M.

Your penis is going to grow during puberty, but you probably won't notice a change in the size of your penis for a while," cautioned Dr. M. "It will grow longer and wider as you get older. But always remember, each boy sees changes at different times during puberty so don't be concerned if your penis grows earlier or later than other boys.

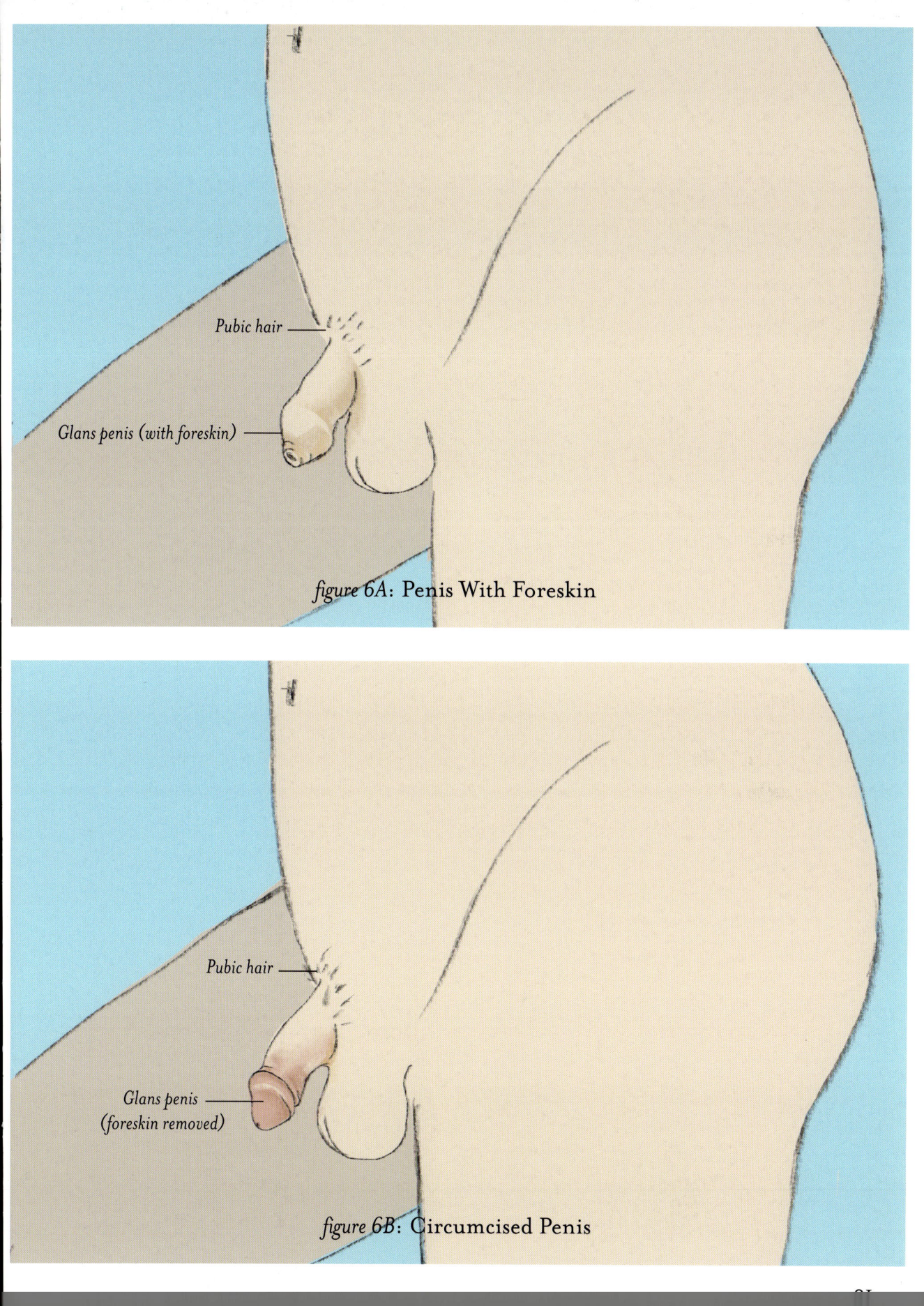

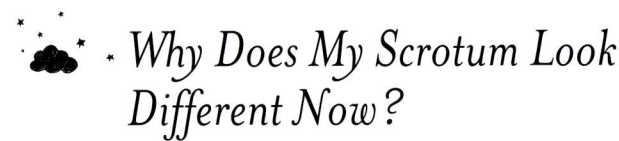 Why Does My Scrotum Look Different Now?

Next, let's talk about the **scrotum**.

You can see in this anatomy figure that the scrotum is a sack of skin that holds two **testicles** (*TESS-tuh-kulls*). Now that you're in puberty, here are some changes to look for in the scrotum.

"You were right when you thought your scrotum was getting bigger, Will," said Dr. M. "During early puberty, this is normal. The scrotum also becomes darker with small bumps. The bumps are where pubic hair is going to grow."

"At the same time that changes are happening in the scrotum, the testicles inside the scrotum are growing. This is why the scrotum is getting larger," explained Dr. M.

Now that we have talked about the penis and scrotum, let's learn about the male reproductive structures that are inside the pelvic cavity.

Dr. M Says:

"The genitals are the penis and scrotum. The inside of the penis looks like a sponge with a tube in the center called the urethra. Urine (pee) flows down the urethra and out the urethral opening. If the foreskin on the glans penis is removed, the penis is described as circumcised. The penis begins growing a little later in puberty. The scrotum is a sack of skin that holds two testicles. It becomes darker and a little larger during early puberty."

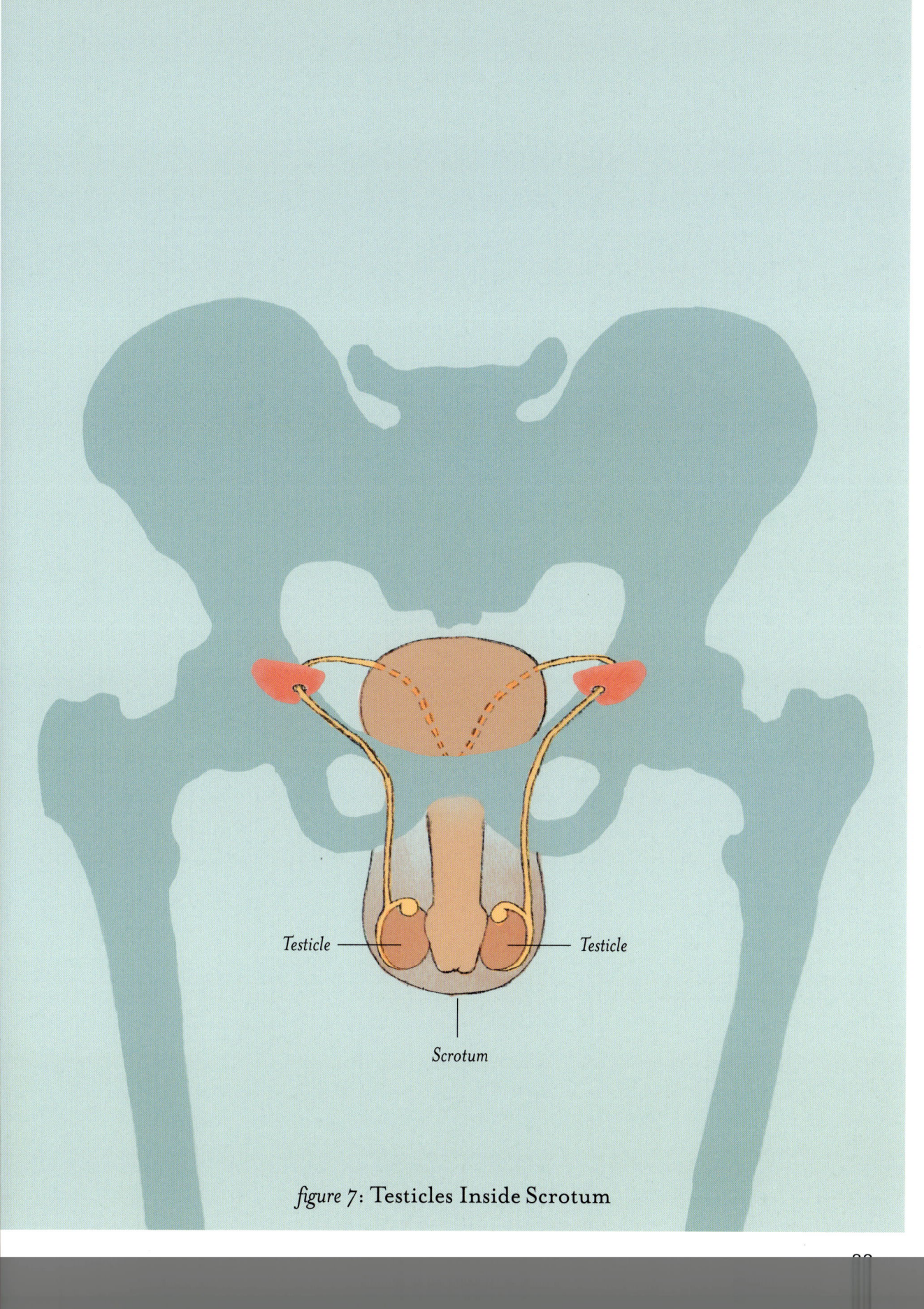

figure 7: Testicles Inside Scrotum

Chapter 4
MAKING SPERM
Where Are Sperm Made?

Your **testicles** are growing because puberty is the time when your testicles start making **sperm**.

Something you might not know about sperm is that they're so small, you need to look at them with a microscope to see them. In fact, if you lined up 500 sperm end-to-end they would make a line that is only one inch long.

The small anatomy figure shows you what a sperm looks like. It has a **head** and a **tail**. Between the head and the tail there is a **middle piece** that contains a small energy source, like a battery. This helps the tail to beat and move the sperm along their journey.

When you become an adult, about 1,000 sperm are made every second.

"So, you see Eric, the testicles become larger because there are so many sperm being produced. And the **scrotum** becomes larger to hold the growing testicles."

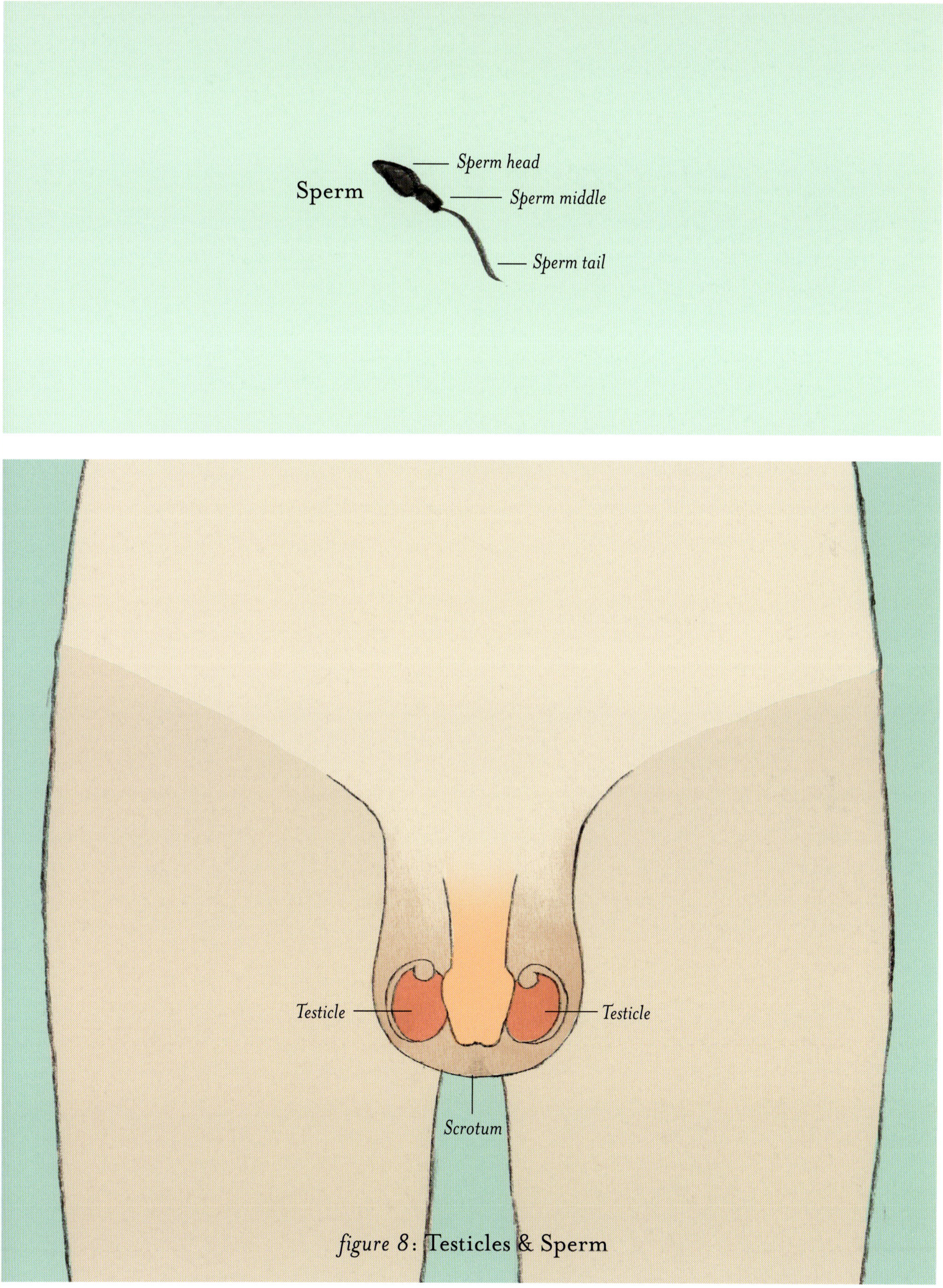

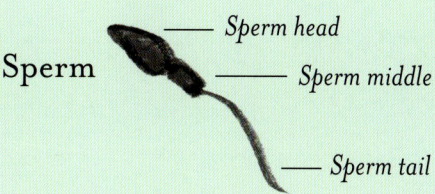

figure 8: Testicles & Sperm

What Happens to My Scrotum When It Gets Hot or Cold?

While sperm are being produced in the **testicles**, they are picky about temperature. They don't like to be very warm or very cold. If the temperature is not right, they begin to die.

The temperature inside your **pelvic cavity** is too warm for sperm and that is why the testicles are hanging inside a sack of skin outside the pelvic cavity in the **scrotum**.

There are small muscles around each testicle that pull the testicles and the scrotum closer to the body to help the sperm stay warm when it is cold outside. The muscles can also relax to let the testicles and the scrotum hang lower when the testicles need to be cooler.

Dr. M Says:

"The testicles grow larger because during puberty they start making 1000 sperm every second. Because the testicles are inside the scrotum, the scrotum also becomes larger."

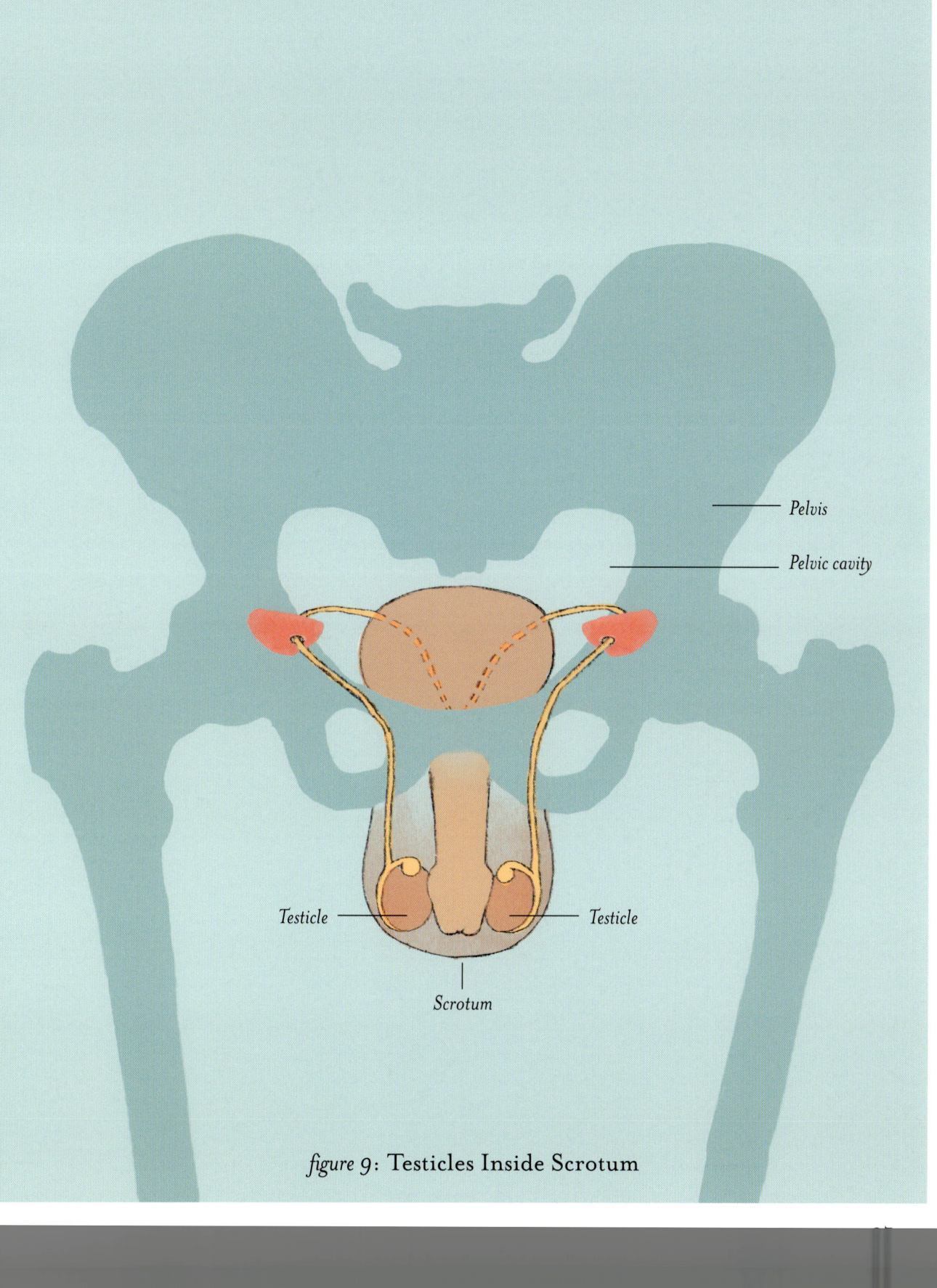

figure 9: Testicles Inside Scrotum

What Is Inside The Testicle?

Let's look inside a **testicle** to see what the sperm-making machinery looks like.

Inside each testicle are several hundred tiny coiled **tubes**. The cells that make sperm are inside these tubes and are waiting patiently for the puberty signal to get going.

When puberty starts, all of the **sperm-making cells** in the tubes begin making sperm at the same time. It is easy to see why the testicles get bigger during puberty.

Also, as you enter puberty, your body makes special chemical substances called **hormones**. Hormones help the tubes in your testicles to make sperm. We'll talk about hormones more next time, but they have truly amazing effects in your body!

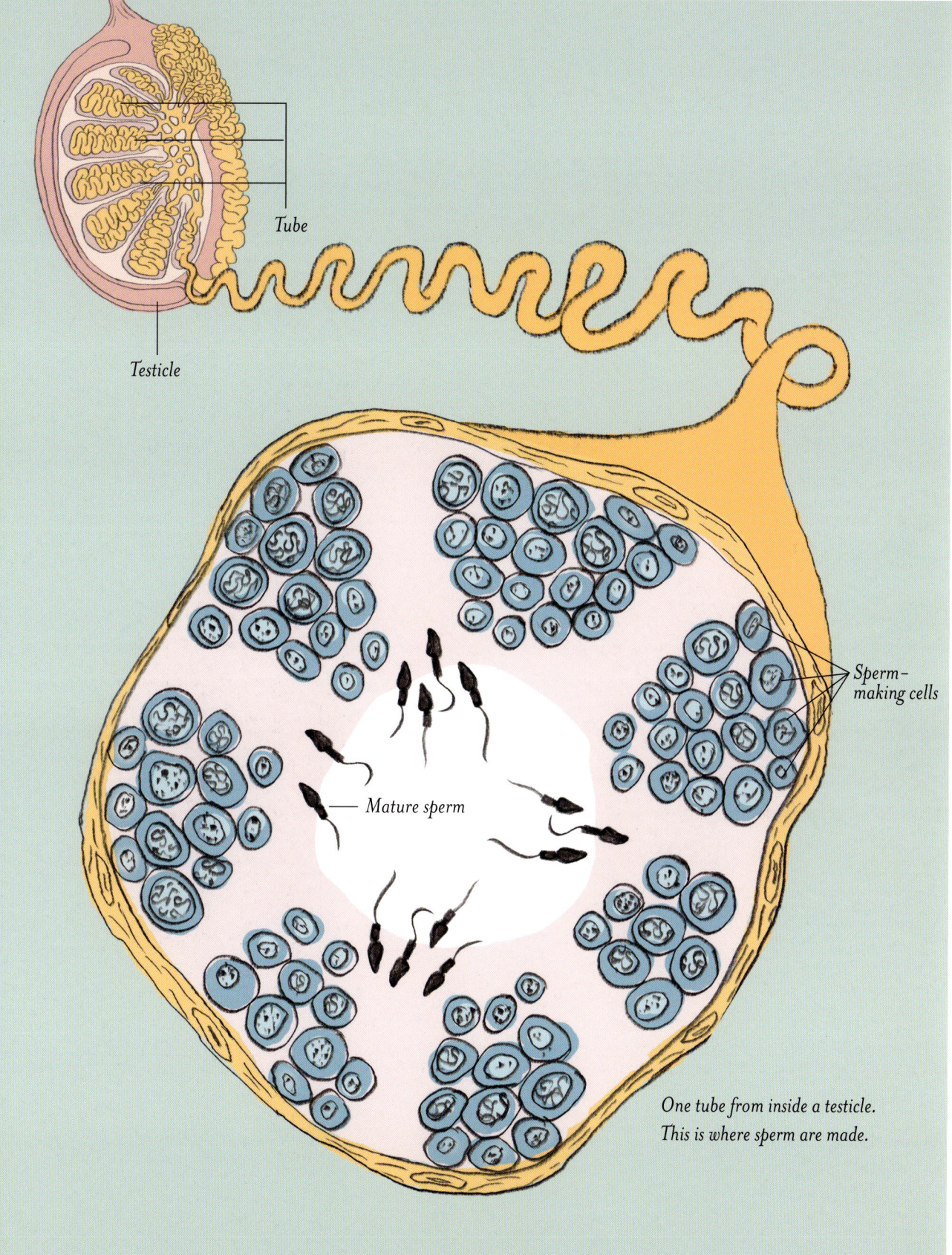

figure 10: Inside a Testicle

Are My Testicles Making Sperm Now?

"Dr. M, are my testicles making sperm now?" asked Ken.

"Yes, your testicles are probably starting the process," said Dr. M.

After you begin puberty, sperm are constantly being produced. A lot more are being made than are needed so most of them die.

There will still be a large number of sperm that do survive and leave the testicles to make a long journey to the penis.

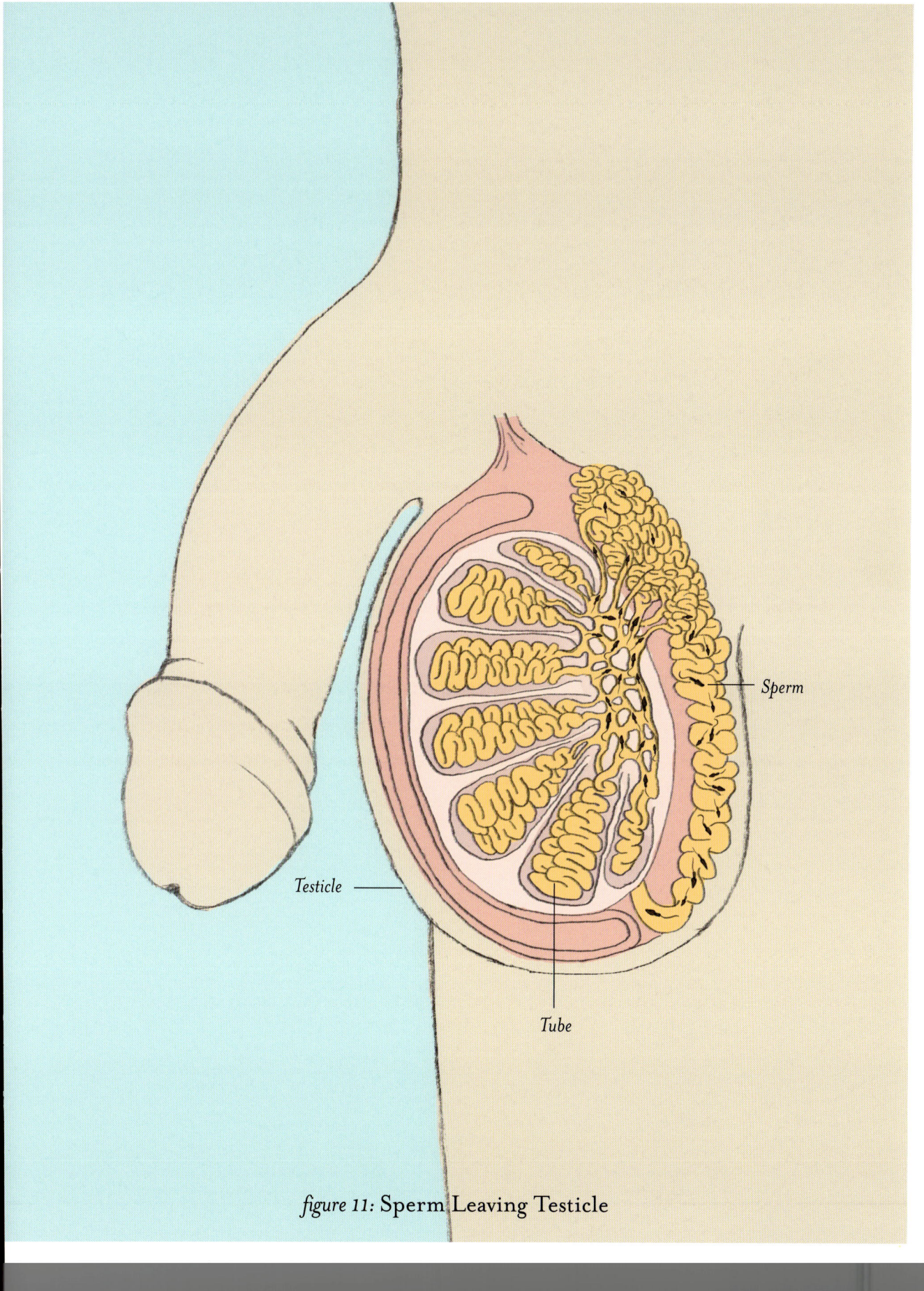

figure 11: Sperm Leaving Testicle

Chapter 5

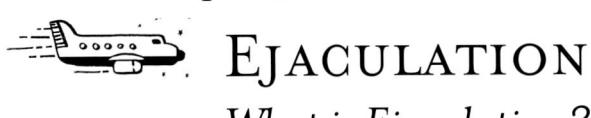 # EJACULATION
What is Ejaculation?

Ken turned to Eric. "I'm confused. How do sperm get from the testicles to the penis?"

Eric looked confused too. "I don't know. Dr. M said something about tubes, but I don't understand what is going on here either."

"Dr. M, we are confused about how sperm get from the testicles to the penis?" said Ken.

"I understand why you are confused," said Dr. M. "What I haven't talked to you about yet is **ejaculation** *(ee-JACK-you-lay-shun)*. Ejaculation is when sperm come out of the urethral opening at the end of the penis."

The way this happens is that sperm are pushed into a long tube called the **vas deferens** *(vas DEF-ur-ins)*. In this anatomy figure, you can see one vas deferens coming out of the right testicle and one coming out of the left testicle.

There are tiny muscles in the wall that forms the vas deferens. The brain tells these little muscles to contract and squeeze the sperm along the tube.

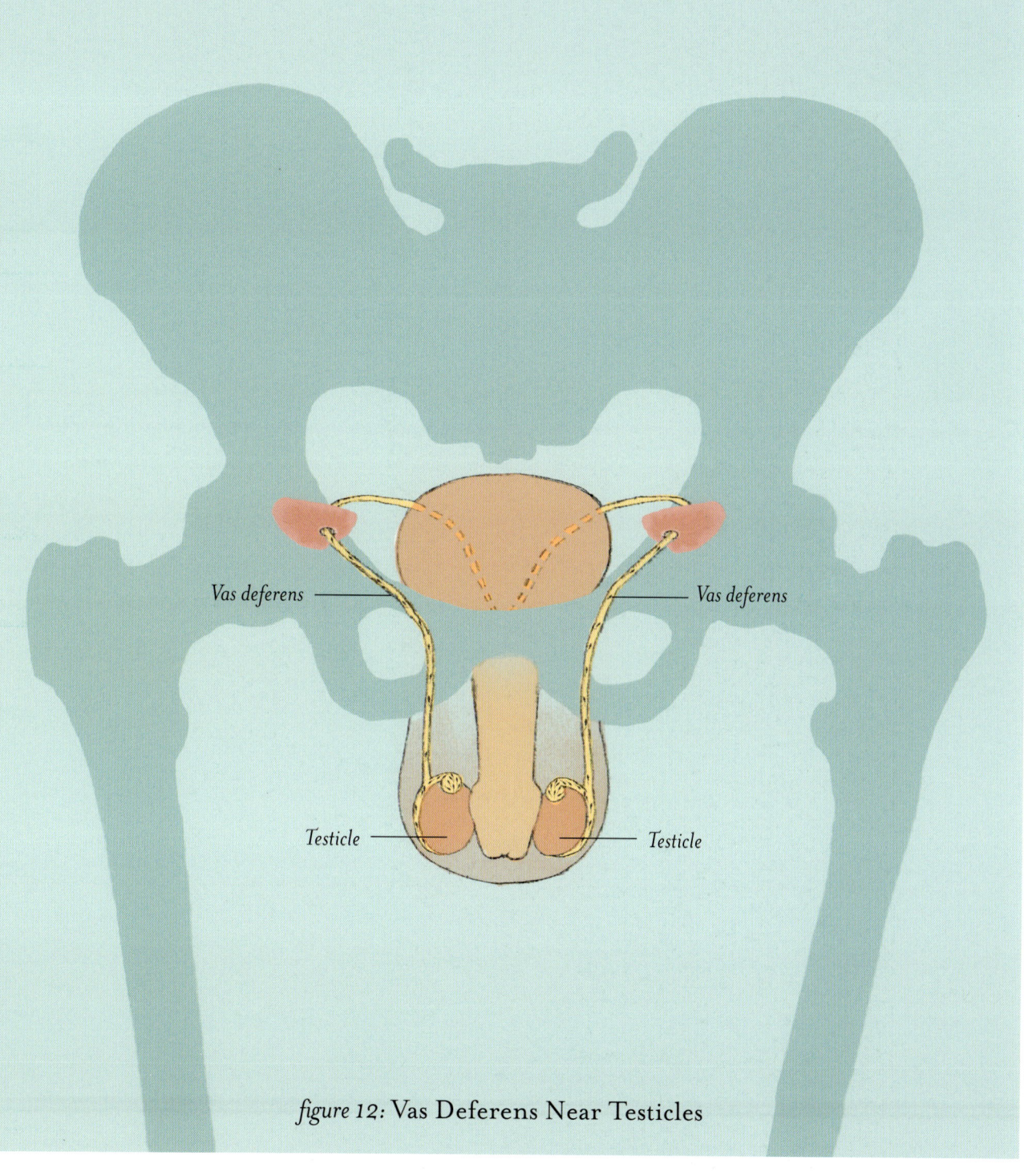

figure 12: Vas Deferens Near Testicles

How Do Sperm Get From the Testicles to the Penis?

The **vas deferens** passes through a small opening in muscle in the abdominal wall and enters the **pelvic cavity**.

"Abdominal wall — is that the same as your six-pack?" asked Will, slapping his stomach.

"Yes, Will," laughed Dr. M. "They are the same."

The vas deferens dives down deep into the pelvic cavity behind a structure that looks like a big balloon. This is the **urinary** *(UR-in-air-ee)* **bladder** where urine is stored until you are ready to pee.

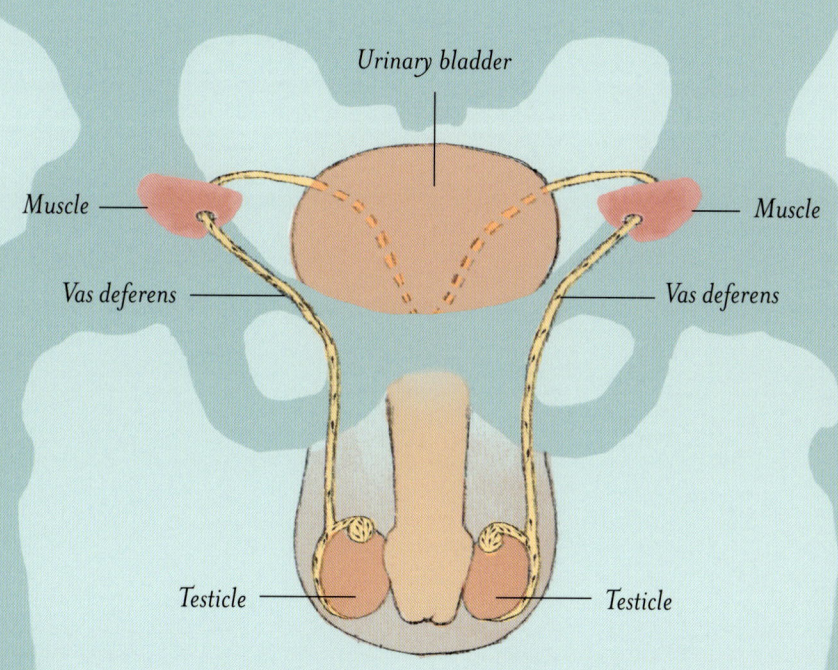

figure 13: Vas Deferens Into Pelvic Cavity

How Do Sperm Get Energy?

Sperm travel a long distance from the testicle to the beginning of the penis. They need nutrients to finish their journey.

Inside the pelvic cavity are two **male glands**, the **seminal vesicles** and the **prostate gland**. They make fluid that is like an energy drink for the sperm.

You can see these male glands in the anatomy figure.

- There are two **seminal** *(SEM-in-ull)* **vesicles** *(VESS-uh-kulls)*, behind the urinary bladder.

- The **prostate** *(PROS-tate)* **gland** wraps around the beginning of the urethra like a donut.

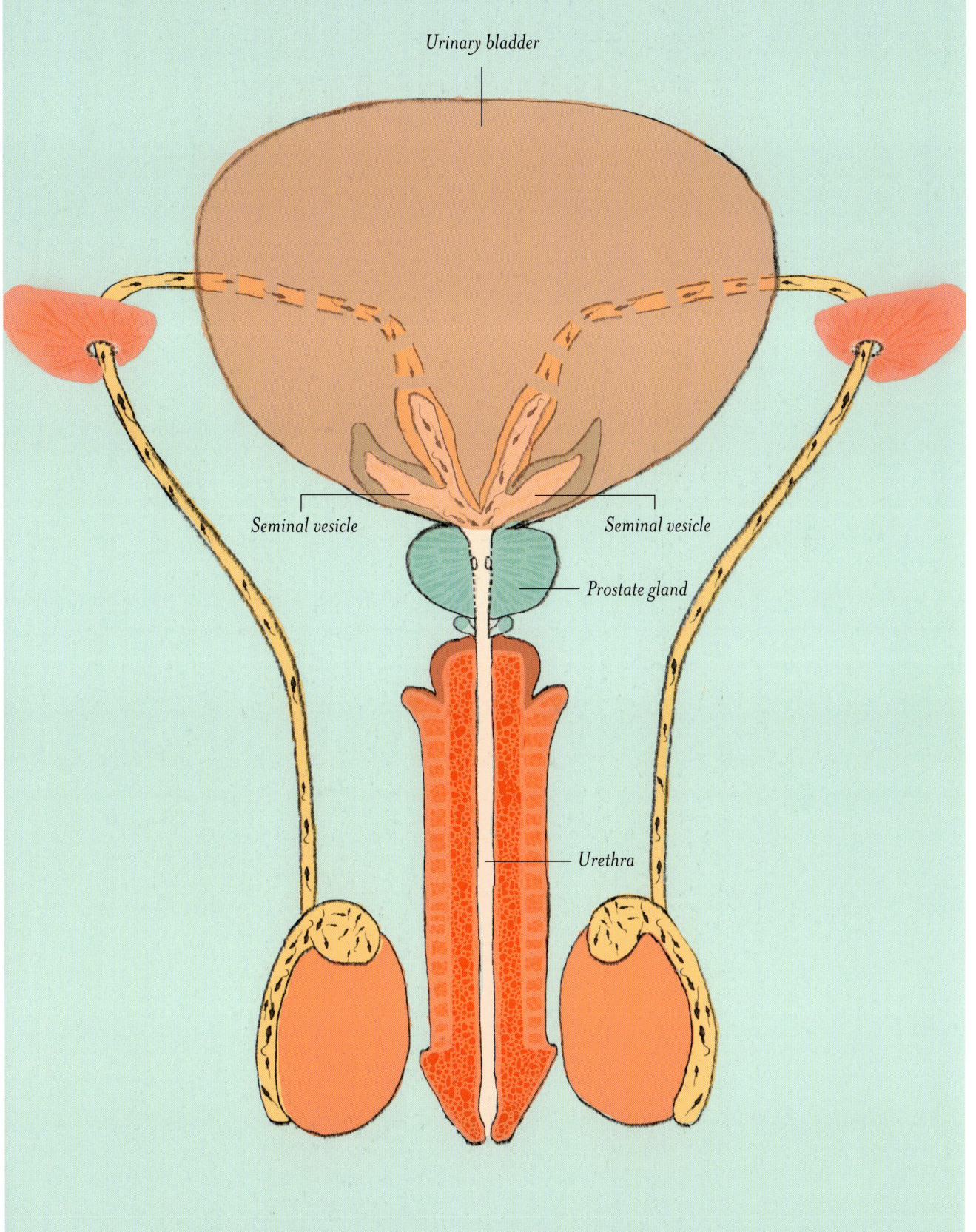

figure 14: Male Glands Inside Pelvic Cavity

What is Semen?

"So, the male glands are just a pit-stop where the sperm can get some nutrients?" asked Eric.

"That's right, Eric," responded Dr. M. "The fluid from the male glands mixes with the sperm and makes a new fluid called **semen** (SEE-men)."

During an ejaculation, semen flows into the **urethra** in the center of the penis and out the end of the penis through the **urethral opening**.

"So, it's not just sperm that comes out the end of the penis during an ejaculation?" asked Ken.

"No, Ken. There is fluid too that is mixed in with the sperm," explained Dr. M. "It's not a lot of fluid. The total amount of fluid plus sperm in one ejaculation is less than one teaspoon."

Dr. M Says:

"Sperm travel inside the vas deferens into the pelvic cavity on their way to the penis. Sperm and fluid from the male glands mix together in the urethra to form semen. Semen comes out the urethral opening at the end of the penis during an ejaculation."

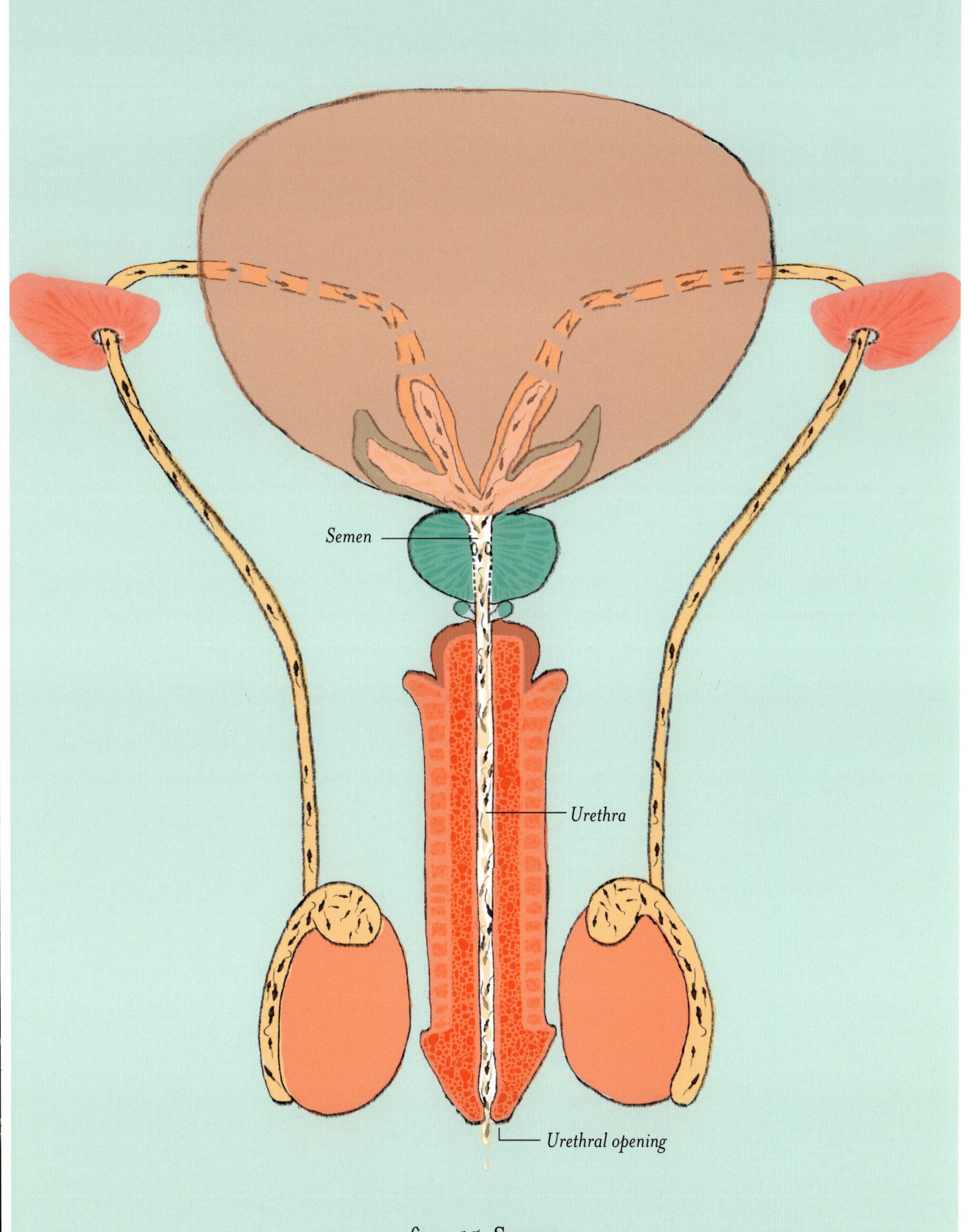

figure 15: Semen

🪐 *Does Semen and Pee Come Out the Same Hole?*

Will turned to the other boys and whispered, "One day I was looking and I saw the hole Dr. M was talking about at the end of my penis. I guess that's the urethral opening, where pee comes out."

Ken whispered back, "She said semen also comes out that hole. Do pee and semen come out at the same time?"

Ken turned to Dr. M. "Hey Dr. M, you said pee comes out the urethral opening. When does semen come out? Do they come out at the same time?"

"No, Ken," answered Dr. M. "Semen and sperm do not come out at the same time."

Normally just pee comes out of the penis. But during an ejaculation, the brain tells the urinary bladder not to let pee come out so only semen will come out of the penis. It actually only takes a few seconds for sperm to get from the testicles to the penis, so an ejaculation does not last very long.

"How can I know when I am going to have an ejaculation? I don't want to be surprised!" asked a concerned Will.

"You don't need to worry," replied Dr. M. "You will know because your brain will tell you before it happens."

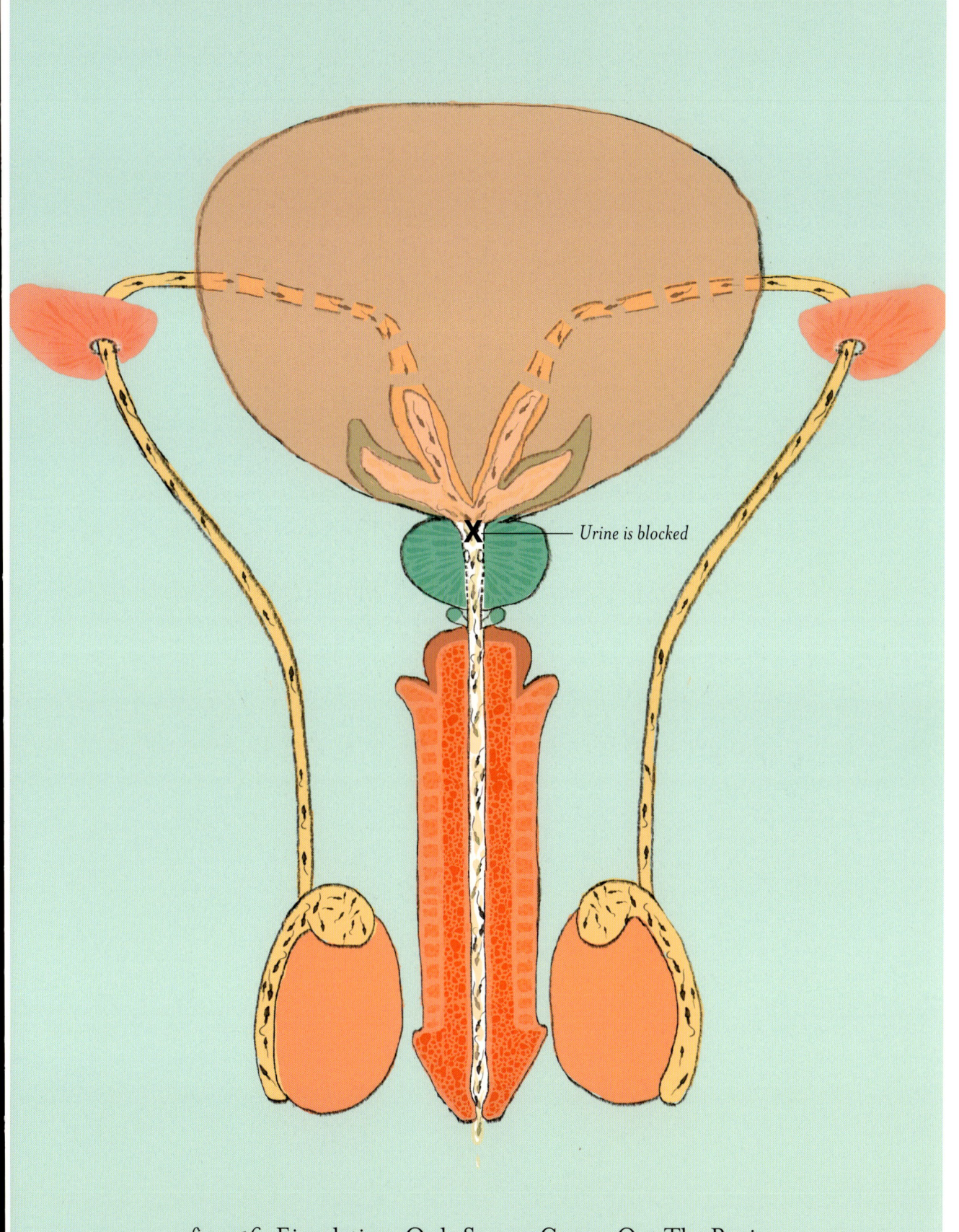

figure 16: Ejaculation-Only Semen Comes Out The Penis

🪐 What's An Adolescent?

It might be interesting for you to know that you are about to become an **adolescent** *(add-uh-LESS-int)*. This is the time between being a child and becoming a young adult. Adolescence lasts many years, into your 20's. During this time, your brain goes through lots of changes that prepare you to live on your own and make your own decisions.

At the beginning of adolescence, while your brain is changing so much, you also start puberty. Hormones guide your body through puberty. They are the reason you notice so many changes in your body like a change in body odor, pimples popping out on your face, and changes in your scrotum.

Puberty only lasts for a few years. By the time you are about 15-16 years old, it will have accomplished its purpose of getting your reproductive structures ready so that you can help make a baby one day.

"Wow! I don't think I know anything about hormones," said Will.

"We can meet again when you notice more changes in your body and learn about hormones," encouraged Dr. M.

"Thanks, Dr. M." said Ken. "It's great to have someone to talk to about all of this stuff. We'll be back to see you soon."

"I look forward to that time!" exclaimed Dr. M.

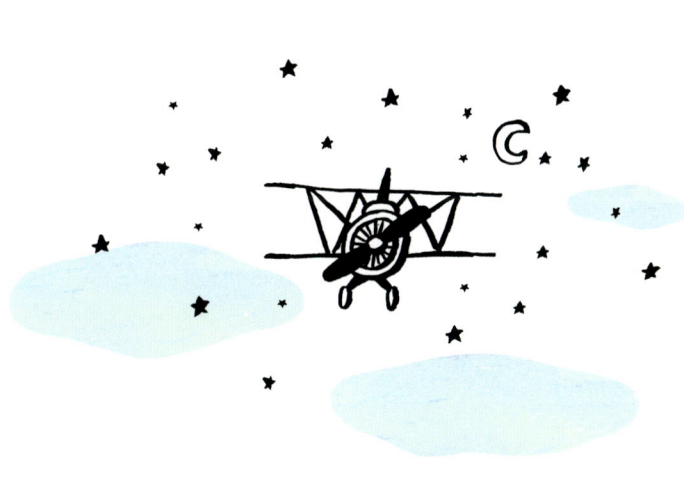

Special Words

Adolescence (add-uh-LESS-ints): the time between being a child and becoming a young adult. You are now an **adolescent** (add-uh-LESS-int). Puberty happens during the first few years of adolescence.

Circumcise (SIR-kum-size): remove the foreskin on the penis

Ejaculation (ee-JACK-you-lay-shun): when semen comes out of the penis

Genitals (JIN-uh-tulls): scrotum and penis

Gland: clump of cells that make a fluid

Hormone: a chemical that travels in the blood and tells cells somewhere else in the body to perform different functions

Pelvis: a circle of bone that surrounds a space called the **pelvic cavity**. Important male reproductive structures like the seminal vesicles and prostate gland are located in the pelvic cavity.

Penis: inside is a **spongy part** that is wrapped around a tube called the urethra. The end of the penis is called the **glans penis**. The glans penis is covered by **foreskin**, also called **prepuce** (PRAY-puce).

Pimples: small lumps in the skin on the face and back that show up during puberty

Prostate (PROS-tate) **gland**: a male gland inside the pelvic cavity that produces nourishment for the sperm and forms part of the semen

Puberty (PEW-bur-tee): prepares your male reproductive structures so you can help make a baby one day. Puberty lasts only a few years during early adolescence.

Pubic (PEW-bic) **hair**: hair that grows near the genitals

Scrotum *(SKRO-tum)*: sack of skin that holds the two testicles

Semen *(SEE-men)*: mixture of sperm plus fluid from the seminal vesicles and prostate gland. Semen comes out of the penis during ejaculation.

Seminal *(SEM-in-ull)* **vesicles** *(VESS-uh-kulls)*: two male glands inside the pelvic cavity that produce nourishment for the sperm and form part of the semen

Sperm: cells produced by **sperm-making cells** in **tubes** in the **testicles**. Sperm help make a baby. The structure of a sperm is **head**, **middle piece**, **tail**.

Testicles *(TESS-tuh-kulls)*: there are two testicles located in the scrotum. Sperm are made in the testicles.

Urinary *(UR-in-air-ee)* **bladder**: stores urine and then sends it down the **urethra** *(you-REE-thruh)* and out the **urethral** *(you-REE-thrull)* **opening** in the penis when you urinate

Vas deferens *(vas DEF-ur-ins)*: sperm travel inside this tube from the testicles to the penis

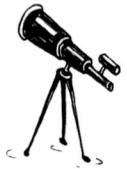

Author
Shelley Metten, M.S., Ph.D.

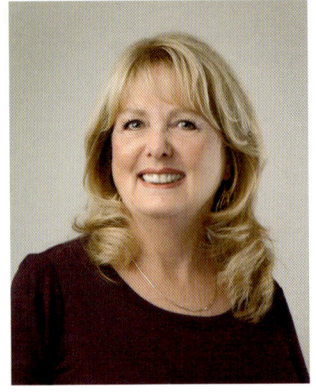

Shelley Metten has been a professor of anatomy at the David Geffen School of Medicine at UCLA for 20 years. Although Dr. Metten enjoys teaching medical students, she has always had a dream to teach children about their bodies. She believes if kids understand how their bodies are put together and function, they will have the wisdom to make good health choices. Her area of expertise is the reproductive system and so it is particularly important to her that girls and boys have an understanding about how their reproductive system changes during puberty.

Dr. Metten has designed the Anatomy for Kids® series with a dual focus: motivating children and supporting parents. The content of the books is age-appropriate and common threads of knowledge are built from one book to the next. Beginning with a young child's first question about where babies come from until your adolescent has reached sexual maturity, Dr. Metten supports parents through Website resources as well as videos and blogs posted on YouTube and Facebook.

Dr. Metten married her high school sweetheart, Greg, and they have two married children and seven young grandchildren. The questions asked by her adorable grandchildren are a daily reminder of the importance of making her dream a reality for all kids.

Co-Author
Alan Estridge

Alan Estridge is a writer, artist, husband, and father. He is also an alumnus of the Animation MFA program at UCLA. The Anatomy for Kids series enables him to bring together a background in biology with a lifelong interest in children's books to relate knowledge in a way that is accessible for all ages.

Design and Illustration

This book is designed under the creative direction of Chris Do, founder of the The Futur and Blind, Inc.

Design and anatomical illustrations by Jessie Do.
Cover illustration by Maggie Chiang.
Dr. M illustration on page 6 by Karen Wang.

Academic and Professional Contributions

Carmine D. Clemente, A.B., M.S., Ph.D., Dr. H.L.	Distinguished Professor of Anatomy and Cell Biology and Professor of Neurobiology, Emeritus David Geffen School of Medicine at UCLA Professor of Surgery (Anatomy) Charles R. Drew University of Medicine and Science Los Angeles, California
Alice Cruz, M.D.	Internal Medicine Cedar-Sinai Medical Group Los Angeles, California
William P. Melega, Ph.D.	Professor, Department of Molecular and Medical Pharmacology David Geffen School of Medicine at UCLA
S. Andrew Schwartz, M.D.	Associate Professor, Department of Orthopaedic Surgery David Geffen School of Medicine at UCLA
Nancy Wayne, Ph.D.	Professor, Department of Physiology David Geffen School of Medicine at UCLA
Shahram Yazdani, M.D.	Professor, Department of Pediatrics David Geffen School of Medicine at UCLA

Special Thank You

Co-Author   Alan Estridge is a person of inspiration, tremendous creative talent and a very dear friend.

Junior Editors   Jonathan Cummings, Shervin Yazdani, Nima Yazdani

Blind   Chris Do is the Founder and Strategic Director of Blind. He has inspired me to think like a storyteller and develop a larger vision for myself as a communicator and author. Also, a special thank you to Jessie Do, the anatomy illustrator and collaborator in the production of this book. Her talent and creative expertise have been the visual foundation of the book.

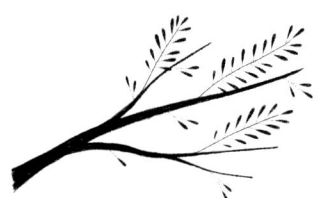